Alkaline Diet

The Best Alkaline Meal Plan To Reduce Body Acid

Barbara Williams

Table of Contents

Introduction

The Alkaline Diet helps you to eat healthy, stay healthy and live your life the way you should. It consists of useful information about the best alkaline meal plan to help you reduce body acids that cause illnesses and diseases.

The Alkaline Diet is both a preventative and curative diet, because it prevents many illnesses and diseases while reversing any health conditions that arise when acid-forming foods are consumed in excess. An acidic body creates an environment which encourages many illnesses and diseases to develop.

The body communicates when things go wrong and in case of excess acidity, there is pain, discomfort, acid influx and other signs and symptoms. Waiting until you fall sick to correct your diet is not the way to go. You need to be proactive and take charge of your life by consuming a well-balanced Alkaline Diet that will ensure that you are healthy at all times.

Many people consume a high quantity of acid-forming foods everyday instead of alkaline forming foods because that is what they are used to. Eating more of what the body needs and less of what it does not need is the only way to become healthy. The Alkaline Diet is made up of a wide variety of nutritious foods that you will enjoy. The foods are tasty whether they are consumed raw or cooked. You will find these foods everywhere you go. You can mix different flavors and colors to create your own recipes that you enjoy. You can also search for recipes that use more alkaline-forming foods than acid-forming foods.

There are many things you will notice, when you start consuming the Alkaline Diet. You will be more energetic to handle the things that you are passionate about. You will regain your health and vitality as the body starts healing and you will live a happy life.

1: Acid-forming Foods vs. Alkaline-forming Foods

All foods are classified as either alkaline-forming foods or acid-forming foods and this depends on the effect they have on our bodies. A food can be sour and acidic like lemon or lime and still have an alkaline effect on the body. This can confuse many people who expect acidic foods to have an acidic effect on the body.

The body requires an acid alkaline balance for ultimate health and energy. If this balance is disturbed by eating a lot of foods that cause acidity, it will have a negative effect on the body .There will be discomfort and many diseases like cancer start setting in. Many people today, take a diet that consists of meat, wheat, dairy products, rice, pasta, pastries and other foods which cause acidity in the body.

Degenerative diseases and other health problems start developing when the body becomes overly acidic because of consuming more acid-forming foods and less alkaline-forming foods instead of vice versa. The major cause of many diseases is acidosis or too much acid in the body. We need to be concerned about what we eat because it determines the life we live and how long we live. In fact, the foundation of most health conditions is caused by acidosis but fortunately, it is preventable. These health conditions can be prevented by taking on alkaline diet.

Acidosis causes the cells to have an acidic pH and to lack oxygen. This provides an environment which illnesses and diseases thrive. An alkaline diet reduces the acidity in the body caused by consumption of an acid-forming diet. An alkaline diet is a good protection against cancer, cardiovascular diseases, stroke, kidney diseases, gallstones, anti-inflammatory diseases like osteoarthritis and rheumatoid arthritis and obesity among other diseases and medical conditions.

The Alkaline diet is also known as acid alkaline balance diet, acid alkaline diet or cancer diet. The alkaline diet has the ability to promote optimal health, prevent diseases and even reverse medical conditions which have been caused by acidified body tissue.

All foods are divided into either acid-forming foods or alkaline-forming foods. Our bodies require 20% of the diet to come from acid-forming foods while 80% should come from alkaline-forming foods. We should therefore maintain the 20 to 80 acid to alkaline proportion to have a natural acid alkaline balance in order to remain in good health.

Unfortunately, the lifestyle many people have adopted today is consuming more of the acid-forming foods and less of alkaline-forming foods in their diet which has led to low-grade acidosis or chronic acidosis in many people.

The blood transports nutrients and oxygen to the whole body and then it carries carbon-dioxide and other toxins to the excretory organs which include the kidneys, lungs and skin. Healthy blood creates a healthy body and that is why you should monitor your pH or adopt a healthy lifestyle by consuming an alkaline diet.

The pH of blood is supposed to be approximately 7.4 on average, for you to be healthy, but it should range between 7.37 and 7.43. If the pH level of blood falls below 7.37 or if it rises above 7.43, the cells in the body become sluggish while the body tissue becomes unhealthy and these cannot support optimal human health. Your strength, power and immunity against illnesses and diseases are reduced.

You need to eat an alkaline diet that will reduce the acidity in the blood and in other parts of your body.

2: Acidosis

By now you may be asking yourself, what can I do if I have an acidic body that has caused health problems? You need to understand what acidosis is, the effect it has on the body and how to overcome it.

What is acidosis?

Acidosis is having excessive acid in the body. It is the acidity of the blood and body tissue beyond a certain level. The pH of the blood in the arteries should be 7.35. If it falls below that level then low-grade or chronic acidosis may be experienced and this affects all the cells in the body. Cell activities and their functions become affected by acidosis.

High-calorie processed foods compose the major part of most modern diets today. Our bodies are unable to metabolize these foods properly and as a result cancer, diabetes, heart diseases and other health conditions have become too common. To have a healthier and longer active life you need to eat the alkaline diet which is high in alkaline-forming foods and low in acid-forming foods. This is the effect they have on the body.

An acid-forming diet is comprised of foods that when eaten, form acidic indigestion in the body and this causes the acidosis condition.

The causes of acidosis are:

- eating acid-forming foods

- medications

- chemical toxins

- immune system reactions

- stress

- tobacco intake

- alcohol intake

- medical conditions like diabetes

A diet based on acid-forming foods and less alkaline-promoting foods is the main culprit of acidosis. In fact, about 95% of all cases of acidosis are caused by consumption of acid-forming diets.

Body cells and tissue, organs, the digestive system and the excretory system are all affected by how high or how low pH levels are and this should be checked to avoid health problems.

Today, people are more concerned about convenience than health. They feed on fast foods and processed foods with refined sugar and empty calories that have no nutritional value than taking care of their health in the right away.

French fries, burgers, doughnuts, soft drinks and sandwiches are easy to pick from your favorite hotels, restaurants, food cafes, grocery stores and convenience stores which are all over.

Most of these foods and diets have empty calories deficient of providing the body with nutrients that it needs. Yet we keep consuming them daily. We even pack our fridges with these foods and beverages so we don't have to go far when we need them.

As people eat on the run and combine foods that shouldn't be combined, indigestion becomes a constant problem causing acidosis which affects the cells negatively. The cells become unable to perform their usual functions and that is how sicknesses and diseases set in. They start to neutralize the excess acids while detoxifying them from the body in order to prevent them from entering the vital organs and all this puts a strain on them.

Strained cells cannot perform their functions properly and that is why you should start to eat an alkaline diet immediately.

Acidosis creates an environment that is hostile to the cells, organs, muscles, joints and bones. The cells lose their energy, the immune system is weakened and the body develops conditions and diseases like cancer, obesity, bone diseases like arthritis and osteoporosis. These health conditions may strike suddenly or they may develop slowly as the body becomes more and more acidic.

When cells have low pH and they are deprived of oxygen, this makes bacteria, viruses, molds and fungi to breed in or on the body. We need a healthy alkaline environment for our bodies to function properly. In order to maintain a healthy pH balance, you need to take 80% alkalizing foods and beverages and 20% acid-forming ones.

Most practitioners recommend at least 60:40 to 80:20 ration comprised of alkaline diet mainly. Consuming empty calories depletes the cells of energy that is used to detoxify them. This robs the body of health and energy.

Effects of acidosis

Foods are considered as acid-forming foods due to the effect they have on the body and the acidity they leave after combustion. That is why acidic citrus foods like grapefruits, lemons and limes are regarded as alkaline-promoting foods.

Meat eggs sugar wheat flour products dairy products like milk, poultry, eggs and cheese, caffeine, grains, fruits such as plums, cranberries, prunes and soft drinks are acid-forming foods.

Consuming a diet that is made up of low alkaline and high acidic foods creates an environment that diseases thrive in. Cancer, stroke, heart diseases, kidney problems, nutrient deficiencies and memory loss thrive in an environment that is acidic causing an acidic pH and lack of oxygen. Acidosis causes both these conditions encouraging cancerous cells and other diseased cells to develop.

How to Reduce Body Acids for Better Health

Since we now know the main cause of acidosis and the trouble it causes, we can eliminate it and move towards better health and peak performance whether physically or mentally. The solution is eating an alkaline diet also known as an acid alkaline balance diet. The alkaline diet raises the pH level and provides the body tissue with oxygen overcoming the causes and the effects of acidosis.

The best alkaline diet and meal plan consists of plenty of fresh fruits and vegetables, nuts, seeds and other foods. These provide the body with proteins, good fats, carbohydrates, vitamins and minerals most of which can you can get from fruits and vegetables the way nature intended.
For optimum health, you need to take an alkaline diet that consists of mainly fresh fruits and vegetables. These will provide the body with all the nutrients it needs.

The body needs to be alkaline to start healing. You can reduce the body acid by consuming more alkaline foods so that you can neutralize the acidity. You should continue with this healthy habit until the body can become alkaline, thereby attaining the acid alkaline balance. When you reach this level, the cells and body tissue get the right amount of oxygen, the immune system gets a boost and the body starts healing itself.

Healthy cells have high oxygen content and an alkaline pH level. This can be achieved by adopting a healthy lifestyle of sticking to the alkaline diet. When the body is acidic, it becomes difficult to treat any symptoms of illnesses and diseases because of the acidic environment.

The acidity lowers energy production in the cells and instead of fighting illnesses and diseases and detoxifying the body of toxins with the little energy remaining, the cells are strained to detoxify the excess acids. The body becomes overworked and toxins pile up in the body systems.

As a result, the body becomes fatigue and vulnerable to many kind of diseases. As this process repeats itself, terminal diseases become a threat to life.

Alkaline Diet is the most effective method to raise the pH level. Medications, stress, toxic chemicals and medical conditions prevent treatments from becoming effective because they lower the pH level.
Diseases need 3 things in order to thrive:

- acidity

- low pH below 6.4

- low oxygen

When the body is acidic, the pH drops below 6.4 and there is low oxygen. This allows bacteria, viruses, fungus, yeast, and molds to develop very fast. The immune system becomes compromised, organs malfunction and the acidity deactivates the enzymes which are vital for digestion to take place.

Cancer, Candida, cardiovascular diseases, asthma, high blood pressure, kidney diseases, stroke, osteoporosis, arthritis and other health conditions enjoy such an environment and no amount of medication can stop them from progressing.

The acidity in the body causes conditions like osteoporosis. The body tries to help itself by offloading alkaline minerals like calcium, magnesium and sodium from the muscles, bones and other parts of the body to make an alkaline environment.

This means that, the cells compensate for this acidity by offloading sodium from the stomach and calcium from the bones which leads to the onset of rheumatoid arthritis, osteoarthritis, gout, lupus, fibromyalgia and multiple sclerosis.

Although heredity, chemical toxins, environmental pollution and immune reactions play a part in formation of diseases in the body like mesothelioma lung cancer (caused by inhaling asbestos), they only play a minor role. An acidic diet is the one that plays the major part in development of diseases. You should watch what you eat and adopt an alkaline diet that is rich in vitamins and minerals.

In fact, research has shown that diseases cannot survive in an alkaline body and that is why following an alkaline diet is so important to health, longevity and the quality of life you live. Research has also shown that our bodies cannot fight diseases when we don't have a pH balance.

A low pH not only encourages diseases to thrive, it also makes it impossible for the body to heal itself like nature intended. But nature has the cure we need in form of fresh fruits and vegetables, seeds, nuts and other foods which we can consume especially when they are raw or partially cooked to provide our bodies with vitamins, minerals and nutrients for optimal health.

The standard diet in many diets is acidic. You need to have the right pH balance in the blood, body tissue, lymph, urine and all body fluids. This can be achieved by eating more alkaline-yielding foods and less acid-forming foods.

Try as much as you can to get 1/3 of your diet from fresh fruits and vegetables. You can add alkaline-forming foods such as almonds, apricots, raisins, dates, melon, kiwi, citrus fruits, bananas, celery, tomatoes, cherries, zucchini and other foods. However, you don't have to give up acid-forming foods altogether because you still need 20% of them in your diet. You should limit their intake and avoid empty caloric foods.

Avoid

- Sugar: since it is acid-forming.

- Soft drinks: like soda

- Most grains: wheat, wheat flour, rice, pasta, oats, barley etc.

- Animal proteins: cow's milk, cheese, beef, eggs, chicken, mutton, pork etc.

- Alcohol: because it is toxic to your body cells. Alcohol detoxification takes place in the liver. An acidified body requires all the energy, so it is better to relieve the liver from this work so it can be able to detoxify the acids. Furthermore, you don't want additional toxins which will strain the liver.

- Coffee: because of the caffeine

- Chocolate

Eat

- Fruits

- Vegetables the greener the better

- Nuts: like hazelnuts, almonds, chestnuts, macadamia, pecan

- Seeds: like sesame, flax, pumpkin, chia, sunflower

- Healthy fats and oils: such as flax oil, canola oil, olive oil, coconut oil

- Tofu and tempeh

- Herbs and spices: such as ginger, garlic, mint, basil, thyme, parsley, cinnamon, turmeric, oregano, mustard

- Herbal teas: for detoxification such as clovers, red clover and burdock root and alkaline herbal teas like ginger tea, peppermint, hibiscus and chamomile.

3: The Alkaline Meal Plan

The alkaline meal plan consists of foods that contain strength, power and endurance. Our bodies require about 20% of acid-forming foods in the diet to function properly.

When these foods are properly digested with alkaline-promoting foods, the acid alkaline balance is achieved and maintained leading to our bodies operating at optimal levels. When the food is properly digested the body absorbs the optimum nutrients. This way we attain optimum performance in whatever we do.

However, if this balance is not achieved or maintained and the acidic-foods are not properly digested, the body develops a condition known as low-grade or chronic acidosis.

Improper combination of foods usually leads to indigestion. Carbohydrates which are made up of starches and sugars ferment while the indigested proteins putrefy.

This causes the blood and body tissues to hold the excess acids which have not been digested and as a result, alkaline minerals from bones, muscles and other areas of the body are drained to neutralize the acidity and this compromises our health.

As a result, the cells lose energy and the immune system is compromised making it weaker while health is drained. The immune system is weakened and the acidified cells lose their energy and power to protect our bodies and fight illnesses and diseases naturally.

The muscles, tendons, ligaments, joints, organs, cells and bones give in and conditions and diseases plague our lives. We start getting nutrient deficiencies, joint and bone diseases, colon and digestive problems, damage to muscles, tendons and ligaments among other conditions.
Diseases set in which include:

- heart diseases

- cancer

- osteoporosis

- stroke

- arthritis

- digestive problems

- ligament damage

Your cells need oxygen and energy to perform all the functions that sustain life whether it is digesting the food you eat, eliminating the toxins or circulating the blood, but the acidity in the cells deprive them of performing these functions. The organs become strained to detoxify the body of the acidity.

An alkaline diet can save our bodies from this state and in fact, they can reverse the acid-forming health conditions. When you adopt an acid alkaline balance diet by eating the required quantity of acid-forming foods and a high amount of alkaline foods, you encourage your body to alkalize the acidity by itself. The body cells are strengthened and they make the immune system strong.

A strong immunity keeps us healthy and helps the body to repair, rejuvenate, regenerate and replenish the nerves, muscles, bones, ligaments and the whole body for optimum physical, mental and athletic performance. The body is able to carry out all the biological performance as it was meant to do.

The Body pH balance

Foods and beverages are divided into acidic and alkaline foods. The pH level is measured on a scale and the average pH is 7.0 which is said to be neutral. If any food is below 7.0 it is regarded as acidic. If it is above 7.0 it is alkaline.

You need to know your pH level so that if it is acidic, you can alkalize it by eating more alkaline foods. You can test your pH level at home or in the doctor's office. This is easy and all you need are pH strips, your saliva or urine. Testing saliva is the easiest and it is done 2 hours after eating. Urine can be tested first thing in the morning by dipping the pH strip in a glass with your urine and then checking the color.

Use the colors shown on the instructions page sold together with pH strips, to know what you pH is and keep monitoring it, so that you can reach the acid alkaline balance level.

The pH strips can be bought from chemists or health food stores.

Why is pH balance important?

The pH balance in your body is so important because it:

- prevents illnesses and diseases

- enhances the absorption of vitamins and minerals

- increases body metabolism

- energizes you

- reduces fatigue

- maintains the proper body weight

That is why you need to check your pH and maintain the right level. If you are not able to do that, then consume more alkaline-forming foods and keep doing this. A healthy lifestyle is not as expensive as most people believe.

Eat plenty of seasonal fruits and vegetables like melon and spinach and add more foods in the alkaline diet. Eat raw fruits and vegetables as much as you can. Use them to make juices and smoothies, salads and side dishes. If you have to cook vegetables like kale or broccoli, steam them partially to reap the nutrients.

How to control your pH

When you test your pH level and you find that it is below what your body requires to function properly, you can correct the imbalance.

You can correct the imbalance and maintain your natural pH by:

1. Eating more alkaline foods

2. Monitoring stress

3. Ensuring that your medications don't lower your pH level

4. Avoiding pollution

Eat the Alkaline Diet

If you want to maintain your natural pH balance, you need to follow the acid alkaline balance diet. The optimal alkaline diet should consist of 80% alkaline foods. You need an alkaline meal plan that will raise your pH level if it is on the lower side.

This will mean eating more of the alkaline foods and reducing the acid-forming foods.

We can group the foods as follows:

Highest acidic foods

Chocolate, cheese, homogenized milk, wheat, wheat products, peanuts, walnuts, pasta, pastries, beef, pork, blackberries, cranberries, ice-cream, soft drinks and beer among others.

Lower acidic foods

Coffee, corn, white rice, white and brown sugar, cashews, lima beans, navy beans and pinto beans, oats, lamb, chicken, turkey, potatoes and rhubarb among others.

Least acidic foods

Corn oil, kidney beans and string beans, plums, processed honey, eggs, yoghurt, butter and tea.

Highest alkaline foods

These are lemon, lime, papaya, mango, watermelon, grapefruit, onion, raw spinach, asparagus, broccoli, garlic, herbal teas and olive oil among others.

Lower alkaline foods

Apples, almonds, pears, melon, blueberries, okra, green tea, grapes, kiwis, flaxseed oil, zucchini, beet, celery, green beans, squash, lettuce, sweet potato, dates, figs and maple syrup among others.

Least alkaline foods

These are avocados, oranges, raw honey, bananas, peaches, carrot, cabbage, peas, tofu, amaranth millet, chestnuts, pineapple, quinoa and ginger tea among others.

Reduce Stress

Stress affects the natural pH balance even when you are consuming the right foods. If your pH level is low, you need to reduce stress.

Check your Medications

Some of the medications you may be taking can make the pH balance to become acidic.

Avoid Pollution

Smoking, using plastics to microwave food and eating foods that have been sprayed with pesticides or herbicides can affect the acidity in your systems.

4: The Human Digestive System

The best alkaline meal plan includes a properly combined diet for optimal health. When you understand how digestion takes place and the different functions performed by enzymes that aid digestion, then you can plan the best alkaline meal by combining foods properly.

Digestion starts taking place in the mouth when the food mixes with saliva and it continues in the gut until it is passed as feces or stool. Enzymes like amylases or ptyalin break down complex carbohydrates into simple sugars such as glucose. Lipases split the fats into 3 fatty acids. Peptidases and proteases break down proteins into amino acids.

The human digestive system is composed of the:

- Mouth

- Throat

- Esophagus

- Stomach

- Small intestine

- Large intestine/Colon

- Rectum

- Anus

The food goes through each stage of digestion mixing with different enzymes to convert it into nutrients that the body is able to absorb for energy, cell repair and growth. Enzymes aid in digestion so most of them are secreted in the digestive tract while others are found inside the cells to facilitate cellular survival.

In humans, the main area where digestion takes place is in the mouth, the stomach and the small intestines.

Mouth

The digestive tract starts in the mouth and that is where some of the food is digested. When you take your meal and chew it, you break it down in an easier form that can be swallowed.

As you break down the food and turn it around with your tongue it mixes with the enzymes in the saliva known as amylase which is produced in the salivary glands. There are some foods which are completely digested in the mouth and so when you mix them with foods that are digested elsewhere in the body there is some mix up which causes indigestion. This indigestion leads to discomfort, illnesses and diseases.

The food become easy to swallow as it is chewed and as it mixes with saliva. It becomes a ball-like structure known as bolus that passes through the throat and esophagus where further digestion takes place.

Stomach

The food mixes and gets grinded in the stomach. Most of the digestion takes place in the stomach and that is why the pH here is very acidic. The stomach secretes acid and different enzymes which are powerful to be able to digest many different types of foods. The enzymes are secreted by the cells lining the stomach which facilitate absorption of food into the body so that the body can grow, repair itself and become energetic. The food is broken down into a liquid or paste-like texture as it passes into the small intestine.

Small intestine

Most of the digestion in the human body takes place in the small intestine. The small intestine is composed of the duodenum where the milk is digested, the jejunum and the ileum. The liver secretes bile while the pancreas secretes pancreatic juices into the small intestine, to break down the food further so that the body can absorb and assimilate the nutrients into the blood.

Large intestines

Water and minerals are absorbed in the blood when the ingested food moves into the large intestines. This takes place in the colon.

Anus and Rectum

The feces or stool consisting of waste products passes through the rectum and anus.

5: The Digestive Enzymes

The digestion of carbohydrates and lipids starts taking place in the mouth or oral cavity as it mixes with the amylase and other food enzymes in the saliva. Proteins on the other hand are digested in the stomach.

Mouth

Amylase is produced in the salivary glands and this mixes with food as it is chewed and turned over by the tongue.

Stomach

The stomach is the one that plays a major role in the digestion of food by mixing it, grinding or crushing the food and mixing it with enzymes that help digest the food. Gastric enzymes are secreted in the stomach. Enzymes combine with hormones and other compounds in the digestion process.

These include:

- Pepsin which digests proteins into peptides and amino acids

- Hydrochloric acid produced in the parietal cells which destroys bacteria and viruses in the ingested food

- Mucin secreted by the mucous cells which protects the stomach lining from the acids in the stomach

- Gastrin hormone that is produced by the "G cells" found in the stomach which triggers the production of hydrochloric acid and also the intrinsic factor

- Intrinsic Factor which is formed in the stomach by the parietal cells, binds Vitamin B12 so that it is not destroyed by hydrochloric acid so that it can be

- absorbed in the ileum

- Gastric lipase which together with lingual lipase make up the main acid lapses in digestion. Gastric lipase has a pH of 3-6 level.

Pancreas

Pancreatic juice is produced in the pancreas and it passes to the small intestine through the pancreatic duct. When it reaches the small intestine, it continues the process of digestion before the food passes to the large intestines. Acidity causes pancreatitis.

Bile is formed by the liver and stored in the gall bladder. It passes through the bile duct to aid in the digestion of fats and proteins. Acidic bile causes gallstones, which can be very painful.

Small intestine

The following are digestive enzymes and hormones produced within the duodenum:

- Lactase

- Sucrase

- Maltase

- Erepsin

- Secretin

- Gastric inhibitory peptide

- Motilin

- Cholecystokinin

- Somatostatisin

The digestive enzymes are affected by acidosis and when this happens they become unable to perform their functions and the body metabolism is affected. For the digestive enzymes and hormones to function effectively, you need to start consuming an alkaline diet to reduce body fluids.

6: The Best Alkaline Diet

You can reduce the body acid. If you have cancer, arthritis, heart disease, stroke and other health conditions your body is acidic. The sign of acidity in the body whether it is in the blood or body tissue is the acidosis. The pH level is the determining factor between your health and development of diseases.

When cancer patients are tested, they are found to have extreme pH acidity and depletion of oxygen in the cells which encourages development of the cancerous cells. This can form stomach cancer, colon cancer, liver cancer esophagus cancer, pancreatic cancer and other types of cancers and diseases.

Which are the alkalizing foods?

An alkaline diet is mainly composed of fresh fruits and vegetables, certain low calorific whole grains, nuts, seeds, oils and many other foods which we have listed to make it easy for you to consume them regularly.

Health is wealth as they say. You need to take care of your health and that of your loved ones. Treating a disease is straining financially, physically and mentally. It even creates stress and depression and it affects relationships.

We should take charge of our lives and the lives of our loved ones in order to live happy and productive lives. We can do this first and foremost by consuming the best alkaline diet.

The ideal alkaline diet involves balancing of acidifying foods and alkalizing foods to a ratio of 20:80. The body through its organs like the liver and kidneys neutralizes and eliminates any excess acids from the body. However, even a healthy body has a limit as to how much acid it can neutralize and eliminate through the body systems effectively.

Excessive acidity strains the body systems as they try to detoxify these acids. Naturally, the body is created in a way that it is able to maintain the acid-alkaline balance on its own provided that:

- you consume a well-balanced alkaline diet

- the organs function properly

- excess acidity in the body is avoided

This is one of the ways to remain healthy and energetic naturally. Unfortunately, the main diet in many homes is comprised of foods that cause acidity in the body. These acid-forming foods strain the detoxifying system so they accumulate in the body.

The body mechanisms become overwhelmed with the work of removing excess acids from the body. You need to eat an alkalizing diet that will reverse the acidity and reduce the strain on the organs like the kidneys and the liver.

The following are the high alkaline foods. Raisins and spinach are among the most alkaline foods.

Alkalizing Vegetables

- Beets

- Broccoli

- Carrots

- Cabbage

- Cauliflower

- Celery

- Collard greens

- Cucumber

- Kale

- Lettuce

- Onion

- Peas

- Pepper

- Spinach

- Zucchini

Alkalizing Fruits

- Apples

- Bananas

- Grapes

- Lemon

- Lime

- Melon

- Peach

- Pear

- Orange

- Watermelon

Alkalizing Carbohydrates

- Stevia

- Maple syrup

- Rice syrup

- Fresh corn

- Amaranth

- Wild rice

- Potato skins

Alkalizing Proteins

- Almonds

- Chestnuts

- Goat's milk

- Hazelnuts

- Soybeans

- Tofu

- Tempeh

Alkalizing Herbs and Spices

- Basil

- Cinnamon

- Garlic

- Ginger

- Mustard

- Thyme

Fats

- Olive oil

- Flaxseed oil

- Canola oil

- Avocado

7: The Best Alkaline Foods That Reduce Body Acid

Different parts of the body have different pH levels. The stomach is very acidic. The acid in the stomach is to help it to digest different types of foods. The effect the food has on the body whether acid-forming or alkaline-forming, does not depend on the pH of the food. That is why fruits like lemons and limes which are expected to promote acidity within the body are alkalizing because of the citric acid in them.

The best alkaline meal plan to reduce body acids should include the following alkaline foods.

Almonds

Almond nuts and almond milk are alkaline foods which are among the world's healthiest foods. They are alkalizing foods which you can eat to reduce body acids and maintain a natural pH balance. Almonds lower cholesterol, increase muscle gain and are rich in protein, calcium, dietary fiber and iron. They can be eaten between meals as a snack or used as an ingredient in alkaline meal plan diets. A few almonds are enough to give you these benefits and neutralize the body acids.

For each 100g:

- Protein – 44%

- Calcium – 27%

- Iron – 25%

Asparagus

Asparagus is a top food in the alkaline list that helps to neutralize the acidity on the body. This is grouped among the strongest alkaline foods. It is also packed with vitamins, antioxidants, detoxifying and anti-aging properties.

That is why you should start adding it to your meal plan to gain these benefits and reduce body fluids.

For each 100g:

- Vitamin A - 15%

- Iron – 12%

- Vitamin C – 9%

Avocado

Both avocado and avocado oils are packed with nutritional benefits making it in the top list of super-foods as well as one of the best alkaline foods. Avocados are rich in healthy fats, fiber, Vitamin C, Vitamin A and potassium.

You can substitute avocado oil for acid-forming oils. Avocado supplies the good fats in the diet that fight the bad fats in the body. Make dips or slice the avocado and eat it raw.

For each 100g:

- Fiber - 27%

- Vitamin C - 17%

- Vitamin A - 3%

Basil

Herbs and spices play an important role in making us alkaline by cancelling the effects of acid-promoting foods. Basil is a great alkaline addition to most menus although you may not have known. It is also rich in flavonoids and is a good source of

Vitamin K and Vitamin A. Add basil to your list of alkalizing foods. Vitamin K helps in the clotting of blood.

For each 100g:

- Vitamin K – 345%

- Vitamin A – 175%

- Calcium – 18%

Beetroot

Not only is beetroot alkaline, it has anti-cancerous properties and is a rich source of iron, folate and carotenoids. Many people eat beetroots as a side dish but you can make a healthy juice or smoothie with them. It is an important antioxidant and that is why it fights cancer in the body.

For each 100g:

- Folate - 75%

- Vitamin K - 11%

- Vitamin C - 8%

Broccoli

This is one of the alkaline foods that you should take often because of its nutritional value and its ability to fight and prevent some types of cancers. Broccoli boosts your pH level which in turn reduces acidity in the body.

Many people eat broccoli almost daily but 3-4 times a week is good enough. Steam the broccoli to get the most benefits from it. You can also bake it or use it in the broccoli recipes as a healthy addition to your alkaline meal diet. The high Vitamin C content helps to fight infections and diseases including cancer.

For each 100g:

- Vitamin C - 135%

- Vitamin A - 11%

- Calcium – 4%

Brussels sprouts

Brussels sprouts are healthy vegetables belonging to the same family as broccoli and cauliflower which break down body acids in the body leaving you more alkaline.

For each 100g:

- Vitamin C - 142%

- Vitamin A - 15%

Cabbage

Cabbage is known to fight and prevent cancer and that is why it should be eaten often. In fact, it can reverse some types of cancer especially if it is organically grown. It is low in calories and makes you feel full. It helps in digestion and boosts your pH levels.

You should steam this alkaline vegetable lightly on low heat, leaves it tasting great, while it retains the nutrients which would otherwise be destroyed by too much during cooking. Look for a good recipe for cabbage and you will enjoy it.

For each 100g:

- Vitamin A – 54%

- Calcium – 5%

- Vitamin C – 3%

Carrot

Carrots are rich in Vitamin A, Vitamin C, antioxidants, fiber and potassium. Taking carrots is good for the eyes whether you take it as a juice, smoothie, steamed or when used in salads or chewed raw.

They are alkaline and tasty while they add color to the food. Many people have a good habit of including carrots as part of their diet but what they don't know is that it is one of the best foods to eat because of their vitamin, carotenoid and flavonoid content. Start chewing a raw carrot now and then or include them in your alkaline diet.

For each 100g:

- Vitamin A - 336%

- Vitamin C – 10%

- Calcium – 3%

Cauliflower

Cauliflower is rich in Vitamin C and a non-fruit source of this essential vitamin. It can be steamed or taken raw in salads or smoothies. You can also mix it with other ingredients to make an alkaline diet that fights cancerous diseases and other illnesses and diseases.

For each 100g:

- Vitamin C – 77%

- Calcium – 2%

- Iron – 2%

Celery

This is one of the alkaline foods that you can use to make salads, smoothies or soup whether you like the taste or not. Celery is one of the world's healthiest foods so you get used to eating it often. It is a low-calorific vegetable which is packed with nutrients.

You can use it to make a green smoothie or add it to a fruit smoothie. It is recommended to people with osteoarthritis, rheumatoid arthritis and cancer.

Collard Greens

These strong alkaline vegetables are among the most effective cancer-fighting foods you can find. It is so rich in Vitamin A and other nutrients that you cannot afford to leave it out of your alkaline meal plan.

For each 100g:

- Vitamin A – 230%

- Vitamin C- 20%

- Calcium – 20%

Eggplant

Eggplant is a popular veggie you should always add when you go food shopping. This is one of those foods you are sure to find in many diets. You can eat as many times as you like without worrying about calories. You can eat it several times a day either as a side dish, roasted or cooked with your food to balance the acidity in other foods consumed each day.

Flaxseed and Flax Oil

Taking freshly ground flaxseed or whole seeds as well as cooking with flax oil will help your body to stay alkaline. You can add whole flaxseeds in your meal plan or sprinkle them on food. Try to add them to your smoothies or ingredients when preparing your meals.

For each 100g:

- Calcium – 37%

- Iron – 46%

Garlic

Garlic is a powerhouse of so many nutrients and also a body cleanser used in detoxifying diets. Garlic lowers blood pressure, fights cancer and keeps it off. Adding some cloves of garlic to your green cleansing smoothie or mincing it while cooking is a good habit. Adding garlic to onions while stir-frying your favorite alkaline vegetable adds a great taste to them. Each clove consists of about 2% of Vitamin C. Garlic has anti-bacterial properties so it is used to fight infections.

Ginger

The health benefits of ginger are numerous and people have realized this so they are using it more and more. Ginger is one of the superfoods that you don't want to miss in your alkaline diet. It is alkaline and it has anti-inflammatory and detoxifying properties.

You can mince or grind the fresh garlic when cooking it or make garlic tea. If it is not available you can use powdered garlic.

For each 100g:

- Protein – 44%

- Calcium – 27%

- Iron – 25%

Goat's Milk

Goat's milk is alkaline and it is better than cow's milk by far. Cow's milk is acidic on the body while goat's milk is alkalizing on the body. There are many people who cannot tolerate cow's milk but they have goat milk tolerance.

For each 100g:

- Calcium – 33%

- Vitamin A - 10%

- Vitamin C - 5%

Grapefruit

This is another superfood which you can enjoy. It is one of the most alkaline foods that you should include in your alkaline meal plan. Although it may have an acidic taste, when you consume it, the effect is alkalizing on the body. Grapefruit boosts your body metabolism.
For each 100g:

- Vitamin C – 73%

Green beans

You will find green beans in many grocery stores since they are one of the most popular vegetables used in many household. Green beans are alkaline and low in calories. Preparing and cooking them is quite easy and you can find them in many recipes.

You can enjoy green beans as a side dish, fried or mixed with other ingredients to make stew. They are a good source of Vitamin C, fiber and potassium. You can also get some amount of calcium and iron from them.
For each 100g:

- Vitamin C – 30%

Herbal Teas

The black tea most people are used to taking is acidic on the body. To have an alkalizing effect, you need to start taking and getting used to herbal teas which are available in many food stores.

Herbal teas such as ginger, ginseng, artichoke, hibiscus, chamomile and cinnamon teas among many others do not contain caffeine. They have medicinal benefits which make them popular among users. They are therapeutic and they contain antioxidants and have a pleasant fragrance.

Kale

The health benefits of kale are numerous. Kale is an alkaline food which is a rich source of Vitamin K, Vitamin C, Vitamin A, fiber and a bit of calcium. You should take kale regularly to boost your immune system because of their high Vitamin C content. The Vitamin A they provide is also high for your eyes and other nutritional benefits while Vitamin K helps in the clotting of the blood.

Adding kale leaves (without the hard stem) to your green juice or smoothie, salads or steaming and eating them as a side dish adds value to your meals. You can add the kale to green leafy vegetables like baby spinach and puree them in a blender until smooth.

For each 100g:

- Vitamin A - 206%

- Vitamin C– 134 %

- Calcium – 9%

Kiwi

Kiwi is an alkaline fruit which you can enjoy.

Leeks

Leeks come from the onion family and they are an alkaline food. They rate highly as a pH booster just like onions while they are rich in Vitamin A and Vitamin C. Leeks are popularly used in soups but you can also steam them and add them to other vegetables to take as part of your alkaline diet.

Lemon

Many people believe that lemon is acid-forming because of its acidic taste but this is not so. When lemon is consumed it becomes alkalizing and it puts your pH scale higher up. Lemon is a good source of Vitamin C which neutralizes free radicals.

You should take lemon for protective benefits against infections and some types of cancer like colon cancer. It also helps to detoxify the body of toxins. You should take it regularly by squeezing it in your drinking water, adding a slice to your detoxifying water or using it as an ingredient in your recipes or take it as a lemonade beverage or cocktail, marmalade, jelly or as pickles.

Lemon helps in throat infections, indigestion and constipation, skin care, toothaches, weight-loss, relieves respiratory problems, controls high blood pressure, removes wrinkles, dandruff, corns, old scars and blackheads, sooths toothaches and heals fever and colds.

For each 100g:

- Vitamin C – 51%

Lentils

There are many varieties of lentils which you can add to the table. Lentils are alkaline when you consume them. They are rich in iron, fiber, vitamins, minerals and other nutrients.

Lettuce

Although some people believe lettuce has no nutritional value, it does. By eating it you get an alkaline response in the body. Even if you do not take it for other things, you should eat it for the alkalizing effect it has on the body.

Lima Beans

Lima beans are a good source of iron, calcium and Vitamin C. they are popular among vegetarians and vegans, they are rich in Vitamin C so you can take them even when you are not consuming citrus fruits.

Lime

As much as lime is acidic, it has an alkaline response to the body and it is good to add it to water for detoxification or add it to your green juice or smoothies. Lime raises your pH level when consumed so you should add it to your alkaline meals. Lime has many benefits like assisting digestion, detoxification, weight loss, respiratory problems, skin care, constipation, fever and other conditions. Lime is consumed as a beverage, pickles, jam, jelly and cocktail or in other forms.

Mango

Mangoes are a top food in the alkaline list. This is grouped among the strongest alkaline foods and is also packed with vitamins, antioxidants, detoxifying and anti-aging properties. That is why you should start adding it to your meal plan to gain these benefits.

Melon

Melons are alkaline but you should eat them alone without mixing them with other foods since they pass through the stomach fast. You will see why in later chapters.

Mint

Adding mint to your recipes gives you and your family alkaline advantages. It is good to flavor your food or smoothie with this alkaline-forming food than with acid-forming spices.

Olive Oil

Olive oils have gained popularity for those who care about their health. There is virgin oil and extra virgin oil among other varieties. One Tablespoon of olive oil consists of 9.8g polyunsaturated fat and 1.4g monounsaturated fat.

Onion

Onion is an alkaline food that helps to neutralize the acidity on the body whether it is eaten raw or fried to make food dishes. This is grouped among the strongest alkaline foods and is also packed with vitamins, antioxidants, antibacterial and anti-aging properties. You should eat fresh onions more often because of their alkaline effect.

For each 100g:

- Vitamin C – 17%

Oranges

Oranges are popular fruits and they are among the world healthiest foods. They are packed with healing phytonutrient compounds which are mainly in the peel and white pulp. They are excellent sources of carotenoids and flavonoids. Oranges fight cancer, cardiovascular diseases and prevent kidney stones as well as lowering blood pressure and cholesterol.

The antioxidants in oranges and other foods help to fight free radicals that cause cancer and other diseases. Eating oranges boosts your alkaline level since they are one of the most alkaline foods. They are packed with nature's antioxidants like Vitamin C which fight free radicals in and around cells so they do not destroy DNA and cause diseases like cancer.

They have a high Vitamin C content and you should take them to boost your immune system as long as you don't mix them or other acidic foods like lemon, lime, pineapple, cucumber or grapefruits with your carbohydrates.

The digestion of acidic fruits is different from the digestion of carbohydrates. Oranges are also a good source of fiber, Vitamin A, Vitamin B1, folate, potassium and calcium.

Papaya

Papaya is packed with nature's carotenoids which help the body fight diseases. This is a top food in the alkaline list that helps your body neutralize the acidity caused by consumption of acid-forming foods. Papaya is packed with vitamins, antioxidants and other health benefits. There are different types of papayas which you can enjoy throughout the year.

Parsley

Parsley is used to garnish chicken, steak and other foods. It is an alkaline spice which you should add to your vegetables when you go shopping. You can add it to your blender or juicer when you are preparing juice or smoothie to give it that refreshing taste.

You can grow parsley easily in your garden, pots or containers so you can have it ready and fresh when you need it. Use parsley to garnish your food.

Peas

Peas are a good alkaline food addition to your recipes. You can use them to make stew and other dishes or take them as a side dish. You don't need to add butter to them because they have their own natural taste and the butter makes them acidic.

There are many dishes that you can make using peas. There are also so many stew recipes that you can get. Peas add color to your food.
For each 100g:

- Vitamin C - 97%

- Vitamin A - 22%

Pepper

Pepper whether green, red or yellow are alkaline when eaten and they boost the pH level. You can take eat them raw or you can stir fry them with olive oil, onions and garlic, add them to your recipes or make a vegetable salad. Peppers are a rich source of Vitamin C and other antioxidants and eating them regularly boosts the immune system. To stay alkaline, add peppers to your alkaline diet and you will reap multiple health benefits.

For each 100g:

- Vitamin C - 200%

- Vitamin A - 11 %

Pumpkin

There are many pumpkin recipes which you can use to make colorful alkaline dishes. It is packed with antioxidants that fight diseases like cancer.

For each 100g:

- Vitamin A - 171%

- Vitamin A - 17%

Raisins

The raisins are rich in Vitamin C. These are one of the foods with the highest alkaline content and you should eat them to boost your pH level.

Soybeans

Many people know the health benefits associated with soybeans and soybean products such as tempeh and soy milk. You can substitute meat with tempeh and soy milk with cow's milk if your aim is reducing body acids from your systems.

For each 100g:

- Iron – 162%

- Vitamin C – 19%

- Calcium – 52%

Spinach

If you think of the best sources of alkaline-promoting foods, spinach is one of them. Spinach is among the strongest alkalizing foods that should be added to your diet, especially raw spinach. If you don't like it raw then steam it lightly or stir fry it with onions. Raw spinach can be taken as a salad, a smoothie or juice. Buy baby spinach and put in the blender and add other vegetables like cucumbers, kale, lettuce and celery to make green juice.

For each 100g:

- Vitamin A – 56%

- Vitamin C – 14%

- Iron – 4%

Squash

Just like its counterpart the pumpkin, squash is an important alkaline food packed with vitamins, minerals and antioxidants. The carotenoids in squash and pumpkin give them their color.

Sweet potato

Sweet potatoes which are alkaline in nature are rich in antioxidants which fight diseases like cancer. You can roast, bake, stew or boil sweet potato or use it as an ingredient in many tasty diets.

Instead of cooking potatoes which are acid-forming unless they are cooked with their skin on, incorporate sweet potatoes in your alkaline meal plan. Take them for breakfast instead of acid-forming foods like bread and oats.

They are tasty and even kids like them. Sweet potatoes are available in orange, white, purple and other varieties. You can buy them fresh in many grocery stores and farmers' markets.

For each 100g:

- Vitamin A – 369%

Tomato

Tomatoes are rich in lycopene, Vitamin A, Vitamin C and other carotenoids. You can use tomatoes to make sauce, dips, salads, burgers, sandwiches, smoothies, juices and as an ingredient in many recipes.

Many dishes prepared in many homes use tomatoes as one of the ingredients. There are many varieties of tomatoes which include plum tomatoes, pear tomatoes, cherry tomatoes and grape tomatoes among others.

Watermelon

Watermelon is one of the most alkaline fruits you can enjoy. It is a top food in the alkaline list which helps to neutralize the acidity in your body. This is grouped among the strongest alkaline foods and is also packed with vitamins, antioxidants, detoxifying and anti-aging properties.

If you take them with other foods in one meal they cause fermentation to the other foods that are digested slowly. To gain maximum health benefits eat watermelon and other types of melons alone.

A watermelon juice is colorful and tasty. Cut it into big chunks and puree in a blender or juice extractor, pour into a glass and enjoy. You can take the juice cool or chilly by adding crushed ice cubes when making the juice.

Zucchini

This is an alkaline vegetable that is easy to grow and is also readily available in most grocery stores and farmers' markets. You can steam or bake zucchini or use it in the many recipes available. You can grow zucchini in your garden since they are easy to grow and they take a short time to mature. This way, you can have them fresh when you need them.

The Acid Alkaline Balance Diet

What is the proper pH balance?

Enzymes or biological molecules within the body are usually proteins, although they may be in other forms. What we eat is broken down by enzymes which act as catalysts in the metabolic processes that sustain our lives. Enzymes cause and speed up chemical reactions in the body which include digestion among other functions.

Enzymes are very selective about which chemical reactions they will speed up. In the body, the way the enzymes behave is affected by the pH level in the body tissues and in the blood. That is why it is essential to maintain the right pH levels for a healthier you. If this is not done, the blood or body tissues may cause diseases which could have otherwise been prevented.

The acid alkaline balance diet is therefore crucial to our health and well-being. You need this diet so that the enzymes can digest the foods properly and make the absorption of nutrients into the blood to be transported from one part of the body to another.

The acid alkaline balance diet helps the body metabolism to carry out different functions effectively so that the body eliminates the waste products from the digestive system as it should instead of depositing them in different parts of the body.

The alkaline diet also preserves the sodium, calcium, magnesium and iron in the muscles and bones to prevent them from being offloaded by an alkaline-deficient diet.

This prevents diseases such as arthritis, osteoporosis, multiple sclerosis and lupus. The best alkaline diet promotes health and that is why you should adopt it.

8: Proper Food Combinations

Eating the right foods is important but what your body absorbs and uses depends on whether you have combined the foods properly. You can take the right proportion of acid to alkaline foods but they may ferment in the stomach or putrefy.

For foods to add strength, power and health to our bodies, we need to follow certain proper food combinations. If we do, our bodies will absorb the nutrients as the food passes through the digestive tract.

You will be able to plan the best alkaline diet recipes which you will enjoy.

Avoid eating carbohydrate foods with acidic foods

You should avoid taking carbohydrates such as bread, rice, pasta and potatoes with acidic fruits like oranges, lemons, limes, pineapples, tomatoes and grapefruits. The acid in the fruits destroys the ptyalin which is an enzyme that aids in the digestion of carbohydrates whether they are in form of starch or sugar.

Ptyalin is an enzyme that can only work in an alkaline medium not an acidic medium. What the acid in the sour fruit does is to prevent digestion and encourage fermentation of the carbohydrates within the digestive system.

You can try to eat the fruit 15-30 minutes before you take your meal instead of taking it with breakfast, lunch or dinner. This way, the acid will have cleared the way for the digestion of carbohydrates.

You can also mix tomatoes with leafy vegetables to make salads or smoothies, but never mix them with starchy foods because of their citric, oxalic and malic acid especially when cooked.

Avoid taking proteins with acidic fruits

You should not take proteins such as poultry, beef, fish, eggs, cheese or milk with oranges, pineapples, cucumbers, lemons or grapes. If you want to eat these fruits, eat them alone before meals or take them with fatty proteins like nuts, avocado or others.

The acid in the acidic fruits when consumed with proteins in one meal prevent the gastric acid from flowing into the stomach to digest the proteins. This inhibits digestion and as a result, the proteins putrefy or decompose.

Do not take two concentrated proteins in one meal

Eating two concentrated proteins in one meal overburdens the digestive system. You should not eat meat and cheese, nuts and milk, meat and eggs or other such combinations together. Different proteins require different digestive juices and mixing them delays digestion since their compositions and strength are different. Take one protein in each meal.

Avoid mixing starchy foods with sugars

Many acid fruit sugars need only one hour to be properly digested. If you mix these acid fruit sugars with starchy foods which need two hours to get digested into nutrients or with sweet fruit sugars like dates, figs, cherries, grapes or raisins which take about three hours to pass through the digestive system, then the acid fruit sugars would need to wait for 3 hours and by that time they will have fermented.

The acid would destroy the digestive enzymes needed by the starchy foods so little or no digestion would take place.

Do not take concentrated carbohydrates and concentrated proteins together

The digestion of carbohydrates is different from each other. Carbohydrates (starch and sugar) such as peas, bread, potatoes and cereals use salivary digestion while proteins such as eggs, meat, cheese and nuts use gastric digestion which is acidic. When you consume carbohydrates and proteins in one meal, they mix with each other and both interfere with effective digestion causing indigestion, gas and discomfort among other problems. As a result, there is fermentation.

That is why many people have a problem digesting beans (except green beans) which have both carbohydrate and protein content that requires different digestion processes.

Take milk alone

Do not take milk with other foods like nuts, meat, cheese, cakes or others, take it alone. Milk is digested in the duodenum so when you take it with other foods it inhibits the stomach from secreting the gastric juices necessary for digestion so the food ferments.

Eat melons alone

Melons whether it is watermelon, cantaloupe, pie melon or honeydew melon or any other type should be taken alone. These fruits are digested very fast and so they pass from the stomach within a short time. If you take them with other foods that require more time to be digested, they decompose in the stomach.

Improper digestion in the stomach proceeds to the intestine and that is why it is important to have proper food combinations right from the start.

Why You Should Combine Foods Properly

Taking an alkalizing diet is not enough. You need to combine the foods properly. You need to ensure you that you eat the alkaline balance diet properly. Otherwise, you might fail to achieve the desired pH levels.

When food is properly combined, our bodies gain strength, energy and endurance. Vegetarians and vegans also find the diet useful because of the plant-based foods in the alkaline diet. In fact, it is a well-rounded diet for everyone.

If we combine the foods improperly, we consume empty calories without the nutrients that the body needs. And since the food becomes indigestible or fermented, it can cause various diseases.

This is why we should be careful about what we consume. We should follow an alkaline meal plan that consists of acid alkaline foods and combine them in their right proportions.

Improper combination of foods usually leads to indigestion. Carbohydrates which are made up of starches and sugars ferment while the indigested proteins putrefy.

This cause the blood and body tissues to hold the excess acids which have not been digested and as a result alkaline from bones, muscles and other areas of the body are drained to neutralize the acidity and this comprises our health. As a result, the cells lose energy and the immune system is compromised making it weaker while health is drained.

The immune system is weakened and the acidified cells lose their energy and power to protect our bodies and fight illnesses and diseases. The muscles, tendons, ligaments, joints and bones give in and conditions and diseases plague our lives.

We start getting nutrient deficiencies, joint and bone diseases, colon and digestive problems, damage to muscles, tendons and ligaments among other conditions.

Diseases set in which include:

- heart diseases

- cancer

- osteoporosis

- stroke

- arthritis

- digestive problems

- ligament damage

Your cells need oxygen and energy to perform all the functions that sustain life whether it is digesting the food you eat, eliminating the toxins, etc. But the acidity in the cells deprives them of performing these functions.
When you adopt an acid alkaline diet, you encourage your body to alkalize the acidity.

The body cells are strengthened and they make the immune system strong. A strong immune system fights illnesses and diseases. To have a balanced diet you need good fats also. It is no longer possible to eat a healthy diet without some good fats.

Omega 3 fatty oils contain alpha-linolenic acids which are essential in our bodies.

Plant-based fats:

- avocados

- canola oil

- soybean oil

- nuts

- flaxseed

- linseed

Omega 3 fatty acids are obtained from fatty fish like salmon, sardines, herring, tuna and mackerel. You can also get these essential fatty acids from fish oil, nuts and seeds.

Avocado and olive oil are rich sources of monounsaturated fats and polyunsaturated fats which help us to absorb the lycopene and beta-carotene in vegetables. It is also rich in fiber and folic acid.

What You Need To Change

The average meal consumed in many homes consists of badly combined foods. You may be eating the right foods and wondering why you have indigestion, heartburn, gas and discomfort.
If you combine the foods wrongly the end result will be illnesses and diseases. You may be taking bread and milk, meat and milk, starch and sugar, oats and orange, watermelon with food and similar combinations.

You may be experiencing acid reflux that causes heartburn, coughing and throat irritations. All these can be corrected with an alkaline diet. The stomach acid is eliminated by the alkaline diet.

Today, you will find people consuming all types of foods at the same time. In one day they may take coffee, bread, butter, jam, sauce, ice cream, sandwich, meat, canned fruits, salt, pepper, sugar etc., most of which may be taken in one meal.

The body was not made to digest these combinations at the same time. What happens? There is decomposition of most of these foods which get wasted. Furthermore, they leave a trail of diseases that could have otherwise been avoided.

Many people don't like changing what they are comfortable with but your health is so important. Your health determines the kind of life you will live and this is worth all the effort.

Start by including some of the alkalizing foods in your diet. Make the changes and enjoy the wide range of foods that you have not been eating before. You will notice changes almost immediately. Your immune system will become strong to fight illnesses and diseases. The organs will start functioning properly.

The digestive system will regain its functionality and indigestion, heartburn and constipation will disappear making you feel more comfortable. Your body will start healing and you will be able to do some things you were not able to do before. Your skin, hair, nails, eyes and all internal and external parts of your body will rejuvenate and re-energize. If you are an athlete, you will gain power and endurance to be able to perform at optimal levels.

However, you need to remember to combine foods correctly.

Frequently Asked Questions FAQ

What is the purpose of Alkaline Diet?

It is to neutralize acidity in the body and reverse the health conditions caused by acid-forming foods.

Can I take the Alkaline Diet?

Yes. Everyone needs to take this diet in order to have an acid alkaline balance whether they are sick or not the alkaline diet is curative and preventative.

Do alkaline-forming foods help with acid-reflux?

Yes. Acid-reflux is caused by too much acid in the digestive system. This acid can be neutralized by alkaline-forming foods.

Can the Alkaline Diet help me to lose weight?

Taking the alkaline diet clears waste products and toxins which are held up in the body. They also help in digestion so that any excess fat stored in the body is also eliminated and as you gain health you also lose weight.

You can combine many varieties of alkaline foods especially fresh fruits and vegetables. Take low calorific foods like cabbage, spinach and eggplants which will make you feel full for a long time.

What does cooking do to alkaline foods?

To get optimal benefits you need to eat fruits and vegetables raw but if this does not appeal to your taste buds, you can cook alkaline foods with low heat to preserve the vitamins and minerals.

Use the vegetable broth in other recipes, don't throw it away. Steaming foods helps them to retain the vitamins and minerals. Eat fresh fruits when they are in season when you can get them in plenty. Continue eating them when they are off season by buying them fresh from the farmers' markets.

How about organic foods?

Organic foods may be expensive but they are the best. When foods are grown organically, they have high nutritional value especially since they are grown without the chemical toxins such as pesticides and herbicides. You can buy organic fruits and vegetables from many places.

What is wrong with animal proteins?

Animal proteins like milk, eggs, chicken, beef, sausages, cheese and others contain residues of antibiotics that are used to treat the animal. These are toxins which get into our bodies when we consume animal proteins and they cause diseases.

Conclusion

We have seen how excessive acid-forming foods can cause havoc in our bodies. When we consume too much of these foods and we fail to keep the acid alkaline balance, things go wrong and we suffer from diseases that we could have prevented. Fortunately, the alkaline diet corrects this imbalance and it reverses what went wrong.

You should adopt a healthy lifestyle by consuming the alkaline diet at all times. You may have suffered from chronic diseases for a long time, but an alkaline diet can help you reduce the body acids and regain your health. Maybe you have not fallen sick but you have realized that you have been taking too much acidity into your body.

The time is now, start taking the alkaline diet and combine the foods properly and you will enjoy a good life with a lot of strength, power, vitality and endurance

Made in the USA
San Bernardino, CA
13 July 2016